W9-AXO-072

breathe

simple breathing
techniques
for a calmer,
happier life

jean hall

quadrille

CONTENTS

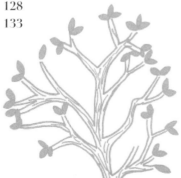

INTRODUCTION

BREATH IS LIFE. It is its very essence – the heart and soul of who we are and it is our constant companion throughout our lifetime. When we are born into this world, the first thing we do is inhale and this signifies the beginning of it all.

Yet, despite the breath being the source of life, most of the time we don't give a second thought to how we breathe and the impact that this has on the way we live.

ALL MOVEMENT FOR LIFE IS CONTAINED WITHIN THE **BREATH**... IT IS THE ORIGINAL TEMPLATE AND INSPIRATION FOR EVERY MOVEMENT

This original blueprint, often referred to as **diaphragmatic breathing**, is the breath at its natural best: full, deep, generous and spacious. Within each in breath there is the opportunity to **open, expand and grow** and with each out breath we have the potential to **release, let go and yield**. Sleeping babes set us the finest example of how to breath, their soft, relaxed bellies gently and rhythmically rising and falling with each in and out breath, respectively.

> ' There is one way of breathing that is shameful and constricted.
>
> Then there is another way: a breath of love that takes you all the way to infinity '
>
> – Rumi

They do this naturally, with no effort. This is perhaps one of the most valuable lessons we can learn: **to let the breath flow naturally, effortlessly and freely**. When they awaken and start moving, their breathing pattern alters to adapt to their new endeavours. Their breathing usually quickens and sharpens a little as their concentration heightens and their body becomes more active and alert. As they tire, their **breathing begins to slow down, helping them to relax and prepare them for rest and sleep**, returning the breath to its fullest depth and ease of the original blueprint.

This natural responsiveness of the breath, which adapts its **pace, rhythm, volume and depth**, supports us through each new and unique situations we find ourselves in and reflects what we are experiencing. **If we feel relaxed, our breathing relaxes**; if we're feeling tight and tense, that's how we will be breathing.

'Breath is the bridge which connects life to consciousness, which unites your body to your thoughts.'

– Thích Nhat Hanh

The breath is a barometer to our internal state of being. It mirrors the mind. What we feel, the breath registers and responds to accordingly.

Into today's high-paced lifestyle, tension often features centre stage, and the body registers this as a threat and begins to operate on 'fight or flight' mode. Whether these tensions are caused by physical situations, mental anxieties or emotional turbulences, the breath's response is to speed up and tighten in an attempt to supply the body and brain with an extra kick of oxygen and energy to cope with the danger it believes it is about to encounter. If stressful thoughts, feelings or situations continue, this response becomes the norm, and we lose touch with our innate ability to return to our **natural original template of full, easy and deep breathing**. We find ourselves stuck in a pattern of perpetual tension.

The good news is that this pattern can be changed. Just as our feelings, thoughts and emotions influence how we breathe, **how we breathe can influence and affect our thoughts and feelings**. In times of turbulence we can turn to the breath to help soothe us, **like the calming waves of the ocean**, so that we may ride the currents of life with a little more ease, grace and steadiness.

By becoming aware and mindful of the breath, **we can allow its flow to return to its natural and full depth**. Allowing, rather than controlling, is essential. Letting, rather than trying to make the breath flow fully and deeply begins to reverse the fight/flight response and informs the body and mind that they are not under threat, so they can relax. **As the breath naturally deepens and softens with mindfulness**, the nervous system rebalances, the heart rate drops, the blood pressure lowers and the whole body and mind calm.

By becoming aware of our breath and receiving its natural flow, **we can transform how we perceive**, think, feel, experience and respond to life. Mindful breathing is the source of it all.

The ancient yogis realised this and they devised a system of deep-breathing practices called *pranayama*, which translates from Sanskrit as 'extension of life energy'. The breathing practices in this book all stem from the yoga tradition and help to return the breath to its natural and optimum pattern that is **full, deep and responsive to life**.

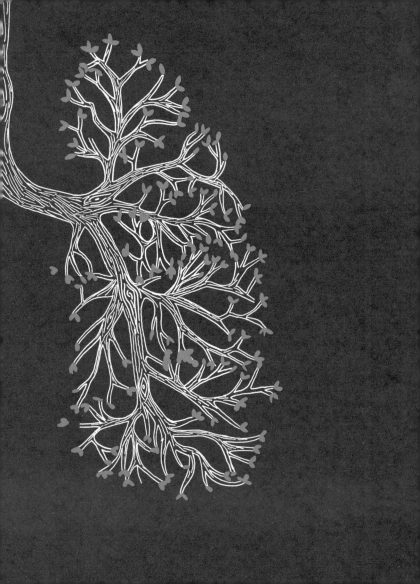

the benefits of breathing well with awareness

Breath is the inspiration and blueprint for all movement in life. When we breathe well, fully and deeply, we can move and be well. Every area of our life is affected by how we breathe, from our physical and mental health to our emotional balance and well-being. The breath's responsiveness and our awareness of it enable us to thrive in life.

THE BENEFITS OF BREATHING WELL WITH AWARENESS

At any given time, the breath has an amazing capacity to respond to and support our changing needs immediately. Although the most efficient way to breathe is diaphragmatically, **our breath is highly sensitive and adapts to life's demands** in each new and different circumstance, responding to everything we experience. When we hear soothing music, see someone we love or a beautiful landscape, **our breathing responds by softening and deepening**. If we hear sad or bad news we are likely to hold our breath, or when we're in an awkward situation, whether emotionally or physically, we tend to tighten the breath.

WHEN WE'RE IN A RUSH THE BREATH **QUICKENS**, AND WHEN WE PANIC THE BREATH **SHORTENS**

WHATEVER WE DO OR FEEL, OUR **BREATH** RESPONDS TO IT

Nurturing our ability to return the breath to its **deep and natural flow** after a challenging experience, for example, when the breath has quickened, is essential to creating healthy breathing. If the breath gets stuck in a particular pattern, it is no longer responsive and supportive to our varied life. **Developing awareness of our breath helps to release our breathing patterns**, so that we can breathe well again.

Breathing well and with mindfulness **empowers our body and enables our mind to be present and calm**. By breathing well and fully we receive generous amounts of oxygen that regenerates our body's cells, nourishes the brain, replenishes the organs and refuels the muscles with the essential nutrients we need in life. Over time, without the **fullness of breath**, the body becomes tired, depleted and stripped of life's energy. We lose our sense of openness, ease and *joie de vivre*.

When we allow the breath to flow deeply and fully through our bodies we begin a chain reaction for positive change and health. **The benefits of breathing mindfully, naturally and deeply are all-encompassing** and support every facet of our mind and body.

WHEN WE BREATHE
DEEPLY AND FULLY:

- **The body relaxes and begins to release tension**, allowing for greater absorption of oxygen into every cell.

- **Oxygen increases within the body**, which creates energy and improves the functionality of all the bodily systems, in particular the circulatory, immune, muscular, endocrine, digestive, nervous and cardiovascular systems.

- **The nervous system is balanced** by the stimulation of the parasympathetic branch. This branch is often referred to as the 'rest and digest' system. It helps to calm and slow the heart rate, conserving energy and enhancing the body's natural ability to heal and recuperate. The parasympathetic systems also improves gastrointestinal activity and this aids healthy digestion, helping to prevent bloating, blockages and other digestive problems.

- **The heart rate lowers**, the muscular system releases tension and the blood vessels are able to dilate, allowing for improved circulation and lowering the body's blood pressure.

- **Oxygen levels flowing to the brain increase**, heightening mental clarity, concentration, stamina and promoting fuller awareness and mindfulness. With increased mindfulness, we are able to notice patterns of tension and behaviour that do not serve us well. These can then be addressed and changed to enhance the relationship we have with ourselves and others.

- **The mind can calm and become focused**, helping to steady and balance and movement so to avoid injury.

- **Pent-up emotion and tension can release**. Next time you're feeling cross, try inhaling and exhaling fully, deeply and slowly several times. You may still feel cross but there will be a little more head space for your mind to calm, the rage to ease and a new perspective to appear. This can also impact on our relationships, helping to cultivate more patience and understanding.

- **Stress hormones are lowered**, in particular adrenalin and cortisol. These hormones are known to suppress the immune system. Through calm, easy breathing the immune system is fortified, which in turn can greatly assist healing and recovery from illness.

- **The mind is harnessed** so that we may be more able to watch our thoughts rather than getting caught up in them. This can help us understand that there is always a different side or perspective. With practice and through awareness, we can develop the ability to guide our thoughts to help self-soothe and heal. This is the foundation of many traditional spiritual practices, which use the body and the breath as the pathway to healing and transformation, helping to develop inner seeing, deeper listening, clearer sensing and greater understanding.

- **The body's production and distribution of natural opiates increases,** helping to strengthen the threshold for pain. This is particularly beneficial for developing natural methods of pain relief and management.

- **Oxygen and carbon dioxide levels are balanced,** which helps to create an alkaline environment and reduces acidity. Inflammation and infection thrive in acidic atmospheres, and so by alkalising the body you help to lessen the risk of infection and inflammation.

'If we live as we breathe,
take in and let go,
we cannot go wrong.'

– Clarissa Pinkola Estes

BREATHING DEEPLY
AND FULLY
FEELS BEAUTIFUL
AND UPLIFTING

THE AMAZING MECHANICS
OF THE BREATH

From the moment we are born, we breathe. It is our biological response to emerging into the world, and best of all, we do it naturally, without being taught how to do it.

When air flows in from the outside, as we breathe in, it is filtered through the network of nasal passages, sinuses, the throat and windpipe before descending into the bronchial branches of the lungs, where oxygen is released and distributed into the bloodstream.

JUST AS THE FORESTS ARE THE LUNGS OF THE EARTH, THE LUNGS ARE LIKE THE FORESTS OF THE BODY.

When we inhale, breath gathers and collects in the lungs, pouring oxygen through the alveoli – the tiny air sacs at the end of the respiratory tree – into the blood stream. At the same time carbon dioxide is drawn from the blood into the lungs and then expelled from the body when we exhale. It is a constant exchange between the outer and inner environments.

JUST AS A BALLOON EXPANDS AND INFLATES
WHEN AIR IS DRAWN INTO IT, SO DO OUR LUNGS –
AND CONSEQUENTLY – THE RIBCAGE.

Just under the lungs is a dome-shaped sheet of
muscle called the diaphragm. It is the core muscle of
respiration, initiating every breath we breathe. The shape
and structure of the diaphragm is like a giant jellyfish
forming a midline within the torso that separates the
thoracic cavity, containing the heart and lungs, from
the abdominal cavity. The tentacles of this jellyfish are
similar to the two tendinous structures, or crura, of the
diaphragm that extend down and attach to the spine.

The movement of the diaphragm is also like a jellyfish.
Imagine the dome-shaped hood of a jellyfish opening
and widening, and then closing and narrowing to propel
itself upwards through the water. Our diaphragm does
the same: as we breathe in, the crura tentacles contract,
drawing the sheet of the diaphragm down towards the
pelvis. This makes space for the lungs to expand, causing
the belly to move outwards. As we breathe out, the crura
relax, which releases the diaphragm to float back up,
pressing on the under surface of the lungs, which in turn
expel the breath and allow the belly to recede.

This steady, constant movement of the diaphragm gently massages the organs within the torso. The ribcage is attached to the spine, which means that with each in breath, the spine is gently lengthened. With each out breath it is released.

THE SPINE AND THE BREATH MOVE TOGETHER

We can often over-emphasise the inhalation, believing that this will ensure we are breathing fully and well. However, it is the exhalation that is crucial for a healthy breath cycle. For example, if we exhale only fifty per cent we can inhale only fifty per cent, leaving us half-breathing. If we breathe out fully, this makes space for the new breath. By allowing the out breath to come to its complete and natural end, we release all of the old breath and the old energy, creating a big open space for the new breath and new energy to flow into and fill.

This will happen naturally if we allow it to and do not interrupt the deep natural flow of our breath. There is no need to make or force the breath to be deeper or fuller. Instead, let it flow out fully and completely and then allow it to flow back, in the same way. We will not need to *take* an in breath, but instead we can *receive* it.

IT IS LIFE'S GIFT TO US
THESE ARE THE TRUE
WORKINGS OF THE BREATH –
TO RECEIVE AND RELEASE ENERGY

In yoga, the inhalation is described as creating rising energy, which is referred to as *prana* and is responsible for growth and renewal. The energetic movement of the inhalation flows upwards from the belly to the chest and is similar to filling up a glass with water. As the water flows into the glass, the water line rises and this is how the in breath can be felt within the body: as rising energy.

On the exhalation *apana* is created, a downward-flowing energy, which is responsible for rooting, grounding and elimination. Again, consider a glass of water that is being emptied. The water flows out from the top of the glass first and then drains through to the bottom with the water line descending. This is the same in the body; as the breath is released on the exhalation, the downward flow can be felt moving and receding from the chest through to the belly. The opposing energies that we find in the breath of rise (prana) and fall (apana) create balance and can be found everywhere in nature – such as summer and winter, day and night, space and earth, movement and stillness.

'Life is in the breath.
He who half-breathes, half-lives.'
– Ancient Proverb

BREATH IN ACTION
– FEELING THE NATURAL MECHANICS OF THE BREATH

1. Lie comfortably on you back with your knees bent, feet on the floor and your hands resting on your belly. Feel the shape and form of your body and let it melt into the ground. Let your thinking mind soften so that you notice your breathing.

2. Inhale deeply and fully through your nose and then exhale through your nose with a soft sigh. Repeat this a couple more times.

3. Now let your natural breathing begin to ease and relax into its own rhythm. Listen and settle into the quietness and simplicity of your breath.

4. Notice how your breath fills your body as you inhale and gently empties as you exhale, like a wave rising and falling. The lungs expand as you breathe in, causing the belly, ribs and chest to rise, and when you exhale, the lungs soften and deflate, causing the chest, ribs and belly to recede and sink.

THE WONDERMENT OF OUR BREATH

🌿 If the lungs were to be unravelled and laid flat they would cover the size of an entire tennis court, about 2,400 km of air pathways.

🌿 The capillaries that surround the alveoli are the smallest blood vessels in human body.

🌿 When we breathe through the nose there are four stages of air filtration (through the nasal hairs, mucous and sinuses and then the throat). But if we breathe through the mouth we omit the first three stages and go straight to stage 4 (nitric oxide). This can result in throat infections such as tonsillitis.

✔ There are about 250 million alveoli (air sacs) in each lung. That's a total of 500 million!

✔ When the brain detects low oxygen levels, it triggers the body to yawn, which releases carbon dioxide from the body so that it can take in a larger amount of oxygen on the next inhalation.

✔ Air contains 21 per cent oxygen but the body only needs 5 per cent. Breathing works more to rid the body of carbon dioxide than to bring in oxygen.

✔ The average person breathes in about of 7 litres of air every minute. That's about 11,000 litres of air every day. This increases fivefold when we are active.

♪ In humans, the size of the left lung is smaller than the right lung. This is to accommodate the heart.

♪ Just by breathing naturally, 70 per cent of our body's waste is removed through our lungs.

♪ Up until a baby is born, its lungs are fluid-filled. When a baby moves through the birth canal the fluid is squeezed out, and at birth the sudden change of temperature and atmosphere triggers the baby's first breath of independent life. This happens about ten seconds after delivery.

- Taste receptors can be found in the lungs, but are only able to detect bitter tastes.

- The left lung has a heart-shaped cavity (cardiac impression) that is created to embrace the heart.

- The lungs are the only human organs that can float on water.

- When the lungs begin to develop in an embryo they can be seen as two little buds growing from the windpipe.

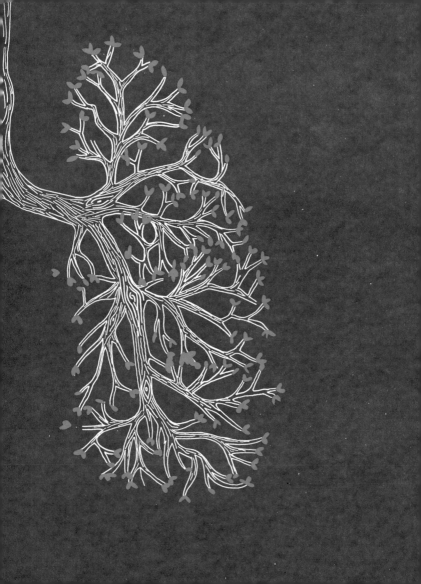

aligning
and
balancing

At the heart of healthy posture lies the balanced alignment of our bones and joints. This helps conduct breath and energy flow and reduces stress and strain throughout the whole body.

BODY, BREATH AND ENERGY

The body is like a container. It contains everything
we are – our energy, our thoughts, our feelings, our
consciousness, our blood, bones, organs and, of course,
our breath.

Like any container, if weak or collapsed, the body will be
compromised and reduced. However, if the container is
constructed well, it will be spacious and strong and has
the capacity wholly to support and store its contents.

If our body is well constructed, aligned and open,
the breath can flow freely, without its energy being
compromised, hindered or leaked away. The body
and breath are intrinsically linked. They support one
another, helping to enhance each other's function.
When both work together in synergy the body and
mind's health, vitality and well-being are increased.
How we position our body can enrich our breath's
flow, and consequently our overall energy for life.

POSTURE

If our posture is poor and the body is collapsed, the ribcage is compressed, which restricts the movement of the diaphragm and reduces the ability of the lungs to expand. This compromises our full and natural breathing, meaning we have less oxygen circulating through our body, which in turn impacts on our energy levels, leaving us feeling tired, lethargic and heavy without being able to support our posture. This lack of postural support in turn leads to further compromised breathing and decreased energy and collapsing of the body. And so it goes on, one affecting the other in a downward spiral. Try this:

- **Slump your posture; round your shoulders forwards and drop your head low**. Notice how you are breathing here. Is the breath shallow or full? Notice your energy. Does it feel lifted and upbeat or heavy and low?

- Now, can you ease out of the slouch by gently breathing in and lengthening your spine? **Breathe out, still feeling your spine long and let your feet open down into the floor** and your shoulders soften and release away from your ears. How does your energy and breath feel now? Notice any changes?

By noticing these changes and shifts, it becomes clear that **how we position our body has a direct affect on our breath** and therefore our energy, our thoughts and our feelings about ourselves and life. It evokes states of being.

By realigning the body out of the collapse of poor posture, we can open up to our full stature and create the space and support for our body's breathing apparatus (lungs, diaphragm, ribs) to function well and fully again. **The breath is more able to flow into areas of the body that are open, easy and free of tension**.

However, sometimes in our keenness to improve our posture we can pull our body into strained positions, leaving us feeling uncomfortable and tense. We may then feel that to make our posture better we need to pull back the shoulders, thrust out the chest, lift up the chin and squeeze in the belly. Yet, as well as feeling unnatural and awkward, this approach to posture realignment creates a lot of unnecessary and negative tension, which tightens and restricts the breath, **blocking the flow of energy** and preventing the body from finding its innate ease and grace. HEALTHY POSTURE ENHANCES...

...OUR SENSE OF SELF, EASE OF BREATH AND ENJOYMENT OF BEING

ALIGNING AND BALANCING

Developing healthy posture does not require so much muscular effort and strength, but rather an awareness of ourselves, and how we are aligning and moving in connection to the ground beneath us. This helps us to become more centred and balanced, which starts from our roots and our foundations.

By rooting into the ground we create a stable foundation from which to grow and expand. **We root in order to rise, and the more we root and yield into the ground,** the more connected we become to gravity, and it is this gravitational pull that helps the body develop its strength and ability to rise. It is gravity that inspires us to stand upright, as our innate response to being pushed is to push back. **Rooting and sensing into the ground** is essential for our growth and postural health.

When sitting or standing let yourself **sense a neutral alignment of your pelvis: that is neither tilted one way or tucked the other.** The bony structure of the pelvis is bowl-like in its shape. This can be a helpful image to imagine when aligning your body in any seated or standing position.

Imagine the bowl of your pelvis positioned upright so none of its contents will spill out over the front, back or sides of its brim. If the pelvic bowl rolls backwards it will cause the back to round and hunch over, which can compress the lungs and internal organs. On the other hand, if the pelvis tilts forwards the belly protrudes, weakening the abdominal muscles and causing the lumbar area of the spine to collapse.

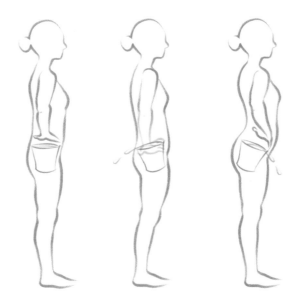

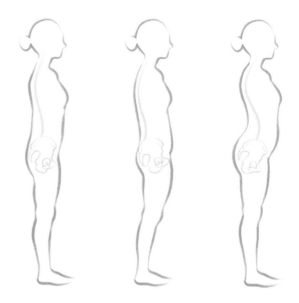

Sensing the pelvis being level will enable the spine to flow upwards, through its natural curves, to the crown of your head. **Balancing this way through the centre of your body will structurally organise you** so that your bones can support your weight and allow your muscles not to overwork in order to establish a healthy posture, which will enhance the flow of breath within.

GUIDELINES FOR LYING

- **Lie down on a comfortable** but firm surface – on a rug or a carpeted floor is ideal. Place a slim book under your head and ease your chin slightly down to create length through the back of your neck.

- Bend your knees and gently hug your legs towards your body, **letting your back soften and open** into the floor.

- Take a few gentle **full breaths** here.

- Now **place and cup your hands over your knees with your fingers pointing down** towards your shins. With your hands still on your knees lengthen your arms straight so that the legs are dangling from your hands, feet and ankles relaxed.

- With your next **out breath release your hands from your knees so that the feet drop to the floor**. Rest your hands on your belly or out to the sides of your body with your palms facing up.

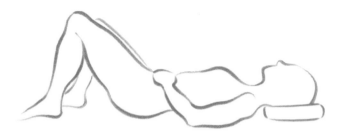

- With your feet hip-width apart, yield them into the floor, **as your knees float into a comfortable balance and alignment with your hips**. Be mindful not to let your knees sway wide.

- **Close your eyes and settle**, letting your whole body release and soften down into the ground. Drop all effort. Surrender to gravity and let go of the need to do anything.

- Rest, be still and **breathe**.

- Remain here for as long as you please (10–15 minutes is optimum), **letting each breath take its time to travel through your whole body** as gravity gently streams through you.

GUIDELINES FOR SITTING

- **Choose a chair to sit on that has a flat and firm surface**. If it is too spongy and soft it will not offer support for the foundation of your seat. To illustrate my point, try standing on cushions or a sofa and you'll soon tire of trying to balance here.

- Sit down and rest your feet on the floor, **breathing softly and easily**.

- Move your attention up your body to your crown. Gently and subtlety move your crown forwards and up, which will lower your chin a little, **lengthening the back of your neck** at the same time.

- **Softly plant your feet down** and move your pelvis into the back of the chair leaving a little space between your back and the chair's back.

- Let your feet feel heavy and your **heels fall into the ground**.

- **Root and anchor through your pelvis**, sensing your sitting bones wide and level on the seat.

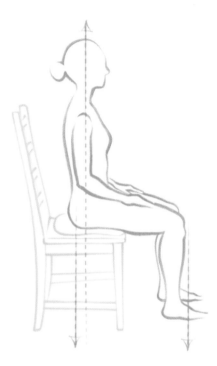

- **Soften** your groin and thighs downwards.

- Easing your crown gently forwards and up, **sense your spine lengthening and aligning** up over the foundation of your pelvis.

- Feel your **collarbones broadening out**, opening your shoulders and chest.

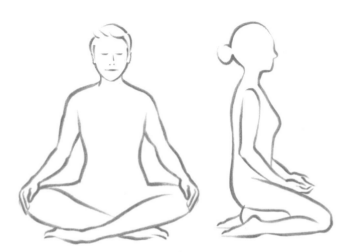

NOTE
These guidelines are also applicable for
sitting cross-legged or on a cushion/bolster.

- **Rest your hands on your lap** with your elbows
  releasing down under your shoulders and your
  shoulders releasing down into your back.

- Relax your facial muscles, gently lowering your eyelids
  until your eyes close.

- As you continue to breathe, feel your pelvis and feet
  softly falling, at the same time as your crown floats.
  With each exhalation **enjoy the length of your spine**.

GUIDELINES FOR STANDING

- **Stand with your feet parallel and hip-width apart**. Soften your knees and spread your weight evenly through both feet. Let the soles open and breathe into the ground with your toes gently spread. Ease your inner arches and anklebones upwards away from the floor. Breathe fully and deeply.

- Sense your body's alignment and line up your pelvis neutrally over your feet, being mindful not to tuck it under or tilt it forwards or backwards. **Let your tailbone release downwards to the floor**.

- **Breathe and sense your spine's length**, gently elongating through the natural curves of your spine and softly raising the crown of your head.

- **Soften your shoulders down** and open your chest while gently lowering your chin and gaze.

- Relax your arms down by the sides of your body and **close your eyes**.

- Be easy and tall, rooted and centred, aware of the space within you and all around you. **Feel your breath's gentle flow, your life source**, in your quiet stillness.

SIMPLE RELAXATION PRACTICES

When we relax we can breathe better, and when we breathe better we feel better, which in turn helps us to breathe better and so it goes. This is because the breath can flow more easily into areas of the body that are relaxed and open.

. . . .

The following relaxation practices are helpful techniques to release tension and reclaim your sense of self. They can be done either seated or lying at any time of the day or night. They can be done at your desk to help give you a mini de-stress session, or, alternatively, at the end of a long, tough day in a quiet, warm and comfortable place. The practices include the gentle touch of our hands to bring awareness to areas of tension and help direct the relaxing and healing flow of breath.

FACIAL RELAXATION

- Start at your eyebrow centre and use your fingers to **softly stroke over them** towards the temples.

- Now intuitively stroke along the contours of your face, **tracing along any lines of tension you are aware of**. You can use both hands with one or two fingers, or you may prefer to use just one hand.

- Follow your instinct and your own awareness as you **breathe and softly stroke away stress** from your face, allowing your expression to relax.

- Finish with your fingers resting just beneath your nose, feeling the warm air of your exhalation against your fingers as you **breathe out**, and the cooler air of your inhalation as you **breathe in**.

EYE PALMING

- Start by **vigorously rubbing your palms** together until they feel hot.

- Close your eyes and gently place the centre of your palms lightly over your eyelids. **Feel the warm darkness soothing and enveloping** your eyes, melting tensions away. Let your breath deepen here.

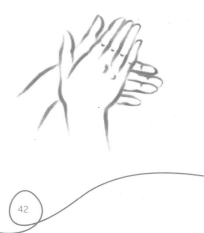

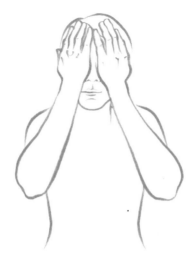

- When you feel ready and still with your palms softly cupped over your eyes, **gently and ever so slightly open your eyelids**, letting the light filter through the cracks between your hands and onto your retinas.

- As your eyes adjust to the light, slowly bring your hands down to rest in your lap and take a few more moments here **breathing softly and evenly**.

TAPPING, STROKING AND SWEEPING

- **Sit, stand or lie in a comfortable position** and bring your right hand to the centre of your left collar bone.

- Using your right hand three centre fingers, **tap along the line of your left collarbone** to the left shoulder.

- Turn your left palm forwards, and still **using your right hand continue to tap down** and along the inside of the left upper and then lower arm, over the inner wrist and into the palm.

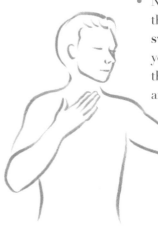

- Now turn the left palm down and with the palm of your right hand **softly sweep and stroke over the back** of your left hand up along the lower and then upper left arm, onto the shoulder and over onto the upper chest.

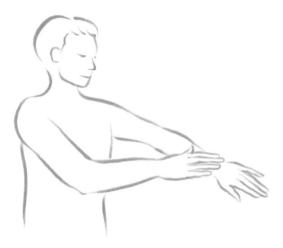

- Rest your right palm on the centre of the chest for a few breaths and then **release the right arm down**.

- Now repeat on the other side, **using your left hand to tap over the right collarbone**, shoulder and down along the inside of the right arm and palm. Then, still using the left hand, sweep over the back of the right hand and up along the right arm onto the chest.

- Rest your left palm on the centre of your chest for a few breaths and release the arm down. **Notice the sensation** across the chest, shoulders and arms.

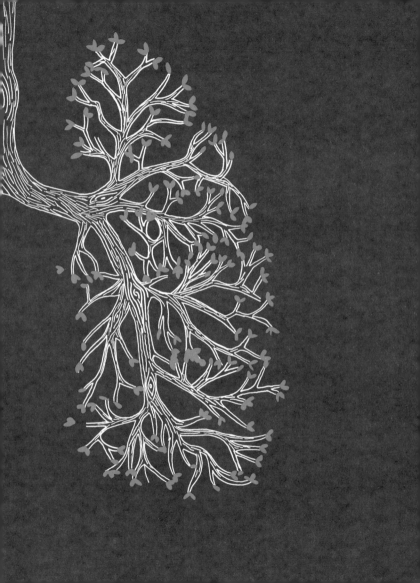

supine practices

The supine practices offer support to the entire body helping to release tension, fatigue and restore energy. They are ideal for tired bodies and particularly aching backs and are an effective way to wind down after a busy day and to help relax the body and mind for a deep and restful night's sleep. Have a look at page 31 for guidelines on how to prepare the body and get comfortable for these supines breathing practices.

SIMPLE BREATH AWARENESS

Throughout most of our day, we tend not to notice our breath – despite it being the source of life. Like a good friend it is always there, and when we give it kindness and attention we can enjoy a richer relationship with it. When we lie down in a relaxed position, it is easier to notice the breath's movement. All we need to do is be aware of it.

1. On a soft but firm surface, lie down on your back in a comfortable position, as described on page 34. Bend your knees and place your feet on the floor hip-width apart, a foot or so from your buttocks. Move your heels so they are a little wider than your toes and gently sway your knees towards each other. **Let your feet root into the floor.** You might prefer to relax your legs down, with your little toes dropping out to the sides.

2. **Take time to get comfortable.** Close your eyes and rest your hands on your belly, beneath the navel or alongside your body, palms facing up. Settle here and soften your body, sensing its weight yield to the floor.

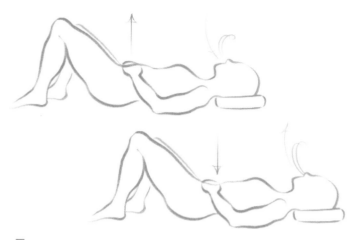

3. Become aware of your breath, without trying to change or improve it. How does your breath feel? Is it short or long, fluid or jerky? **Let your breath be and allow yourself the space and time to listen.**

4. As you listen to your breath, let it naturally soften and deepen, finding its own rhythm. **Enjoy the natural flow, befriending it and immersing your whole being into your breathing.** This simple, conscious act will nurture the friendship and enable you to take refuge in it whenever you want.

Making friends with your breath can be done anywhere – lying down, sitting, standing or walking. The key is to quieten and soften your mind as this makes it easier to listen and hear.

NATURAL DIAPHRAGMATIC BREATH: PART 1

Also known as natural deep breathing, diaphragmatic breathing delivers more oxygen and nourishment to the body than restricted breathing, which is something we tend to do. It soothes the nervous system and strokes the brainwaves, helping to balance our whole being. The natural rhythmic movement of the diaphragm gently massages the internal organs.

1. **Lie on your front with your head to one side.** Rest your arms either side of your head, hands close to the crown.

2. Take a few moments to settle and get comfortable. Relax and soften your facial muscles, let your eyes close and become aware of your breath. **Let your whole body melt into the floor as you exhale.**

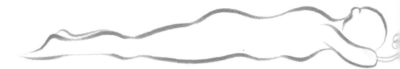

3. **As you inhale fully,** notice how your belly softly presses down into the ground and as you exhale, the belly gently retracts again.

4. As you breathe slowly and naturally, **move your attention to your ribcage and notice how the side ribs move,** widening as you inhale and drawing back as you exhale. Just notice this movement and allow it to be easy without changing it.

5. Widen your attention to your lower back. Feel how it expands and opens as you **breathe in** and softens and releases down as you **breathe out.**

6. **Turn your head to the other side to even out the stretch of your neck** and breathe with the same deep awareness for a few more minutes.

TIP
Imagine your body is an accordion being played by your breath. Drawing open as you inhale, opening and widening your back, ribcage and belly as you receive the breath. Then concertina in as you exhale, receding to release the breath

7. Bring yourself into all fours, **softly spreading your hands and fingers open and feeling your back wide and long**. Have your hands under your shoulders and your knees under your hips. Gently bring your feet together, and as you breathe out, draw your hips back towards your heels. Leave your hands where they are as you ease your buttocks down onto your feet to create a gentle stretch through your spine.

8. **Release your ribs down onto your thighs and lower your chest** and shoulders to bring your arms and forehead to relax down onto the ground. Rest here completely, yielding and surrendering your whole body to gravity.

CLOSE YOUR EYES, SOFTEN AND BREATHE

DEEPENED DIAPHRAGMATIC BREATH: PART 2

This practice evolves from the previous one. It is an expansive practice that helps cultivate a sense of inner spaciousness and stillness as well as connecting us to the natural ebb and flow of the breath.

1. **Gently roll over onto your back.** Bend your knees and place your feet hip-width apart on the floor a few inches from your buttocks. Gently angle your knees in line with your hips and let the soles of your feet release into the floor.

2. Close your eyes and rest your hands on your belly, beneath the navel or alongside your body, palms facing up. **Feel the weight of your body sink into the floor.** Take a few moments to breathe and settle your mind and body.

3. Become aware of your breath and let it spread throughout your body. **Let it melt away the hard edges as you exhale** and gently sense the inner spaces of your body as you inhale.

4. On your next exhalation, **exhale slowly and fully,
letting the breath flow out** and come to its natural
end. Rest here for a moment and feel the gentle pause
at the end of the breath.

5. Soften and let the breath return gently, **like a gentle
wave washing back in shore**, filling the space within
your body.

6. When you sense you are full and the breath has come
to its natural completion, **enjoy the natural pause for
a fleeting moment**, in the open space of that breath.

7. **Let the exhalation begin its flow** and journey out,
releasing, softening and removing the expended energy.

8. When the exhalation is complete, **pause and enjoy
the calm emptiness**.

9. **Receive the new wave of breath gently**, filling and
opening you from the inside.

10. As you continue to breathe like this, notice the
4 naturally occurring stages of each breath.

- **Inhalation and inspiration**
- **Pause in fullness**
- **Exhalation and release**
- **Pause in emptiness**

11. Follow the gentle ebb and flow of the breath
and soften into the gentle pauses between the in and out
breaths. Be mindful not to hold the pauses for too long
but let them be natural and fluid.

12. When you feel ready to close the practice, bend
your knees and softly hug your legs into your torso.
Gently and slowly rock from side to side a few times
and then roll over onto the right side of your body and
make your way up to a sitting position.

SELF-SOOTHING BREATH

The gentle, rhythmic rolling motion in this practice helps soothe the body and the brainwaves. Drawing up the legs and hugging them softly can make powerful feelings be less overwhelming as you protect and contain them with this action.

1. **Come to lie down on your back** in a comfortable position, as described on page 34.

2. Bend your knees up towards your body and gently hug your legs, relaxing your feet and ankles. **Soften and release your shoulders to the floor**, relax your back and lower your chin to lengthen the back of your neck. Let your eyes close.

3. As you hug your legs into your body, bring attention to your breath. Notice its natural rise and fall – **your energy softly rising when you inhale and gently falling when you exhale**. When you inhale, allow your belly and ribs to rise up towards your thighs, then sink back down when you exhale. Settle here for a few moments.

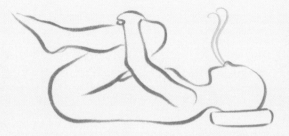

4. Slowly and gently roll your body a little to the
right and then to the left, using the floor to massage
your back. Keep the motion relaxed, soft and rhythmical.

5. **Now begin to coordinate the rocking motion with
your breath**. As you inhale, gently roll to the right, and
as you exhale, roll back to centre. Slowly inhale as you
rock to the left, and exhale as you rock back to centre.

6. Continue rolling for 5–10 minutes, **until you feel
a quiet calm flowing through your body and mind**.
Take time to breathe and move slowly and smoothly.

SIMPLE BREATH RELEASE

This practice helps to release pent-up emotions and tensions from your mind and body.

---

1. **Come to lie down on your back** in a comfortable position, as described on page 34.

2. When you feel comfortable, close your eyes and settle. **Become aware of your body and your breath**, simply noticing them without changing or shifting anything.

- ❧ **How does your body feel?**
- ❧ **Do any areas feel weak or tense?**
- ❧ **Are you breathing through your nose, mouth, or both?**
- ❧ **How does your breathing feel?**
- ❧ **Does it feel tight or relaxed?**
- ❧ **Is it shallow or deep?**

Just notice and listen to each breath. Sometimes simply listening and noticing your breath will enable it to relax. Allow it to flow for a few more moments. **LETTING IT BE**

3. On your next inhalation, **breathe in slowly and fully through your nose**, filling your lungs from the bottom to the top. When you sense you are full, pause and retain the breath for a moment or two.

4. Slowly and completely exhale through your mouth, **sighing your breath away** and letting the weight of your body soften and release into the floor.

5. On your next inhalation, **breathe in slowly and fully again, and pause.** This time hold on to the breath for a little longer but do not strain.

6. Now relax and exhale through your mouth with a long, steady haaaa **sigh, releasing your tensions.**

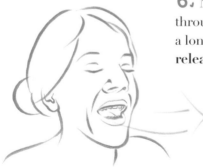

7. On your next inhalation, **breathe in fully and deeply through your nose**, feeling your belly rising, your lungs expanding and your chest opening.

PAUSE WHEN YOU ARE FULL
AT THE TOP OF THE BREATH

8. Slowly and completely exhale through your mouth, sighing **your breath away and letting the weight of your body melt to the ground**, releasing any tension.

9. Repeat this three more times but instead of sighing out, softly purse your lips and blow out through your mouth as **if you are blowing dust from the surface of your mind**. Feel your body sink into the ground with each exhalation.

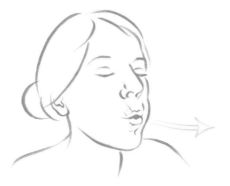

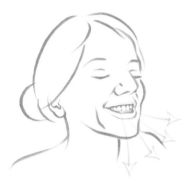

10. Repeat three more times and this time hissss **out through your mouth like an angry snake**, consciously breathing out any irritation, frustration or anger that you maybe feeling.

11. Feel free to repeat any part of this **practice a few more times to release any further tension.**

12. Once you feel a sense of release through your body, heart and mind, **let your breathing relax back to its natural and spontaneous flow.** Fully and slowly exhale each breath before your next inhalation starts its journey through your body. Each time, let your weight soften and fall away into the earth.

MODULATED BREATH
(VILOMA)

Viloma is a foundational breathing practice in Hatha Yoga that helps open and strengthen the lungs, develop concentration and balance the nervous system. Once this basic version has been learned, the breath can be divided further.

1. **Come to lie down on your back** in a comfortable position, as described on page 34.

2. Place your hands on your belly, beneath the navel or alongside your body, **palms facing up**.

3. Close your eyes. **Feel your whole body resting and softening into the floor.** Enjoy a few moments, letting your breathing settle into a slow and rhythmic flow.

4. As you inhale, become aware of how your belly rises as the **breath moves into the lower part of your lungs and gently floods into the upper part**, as your chest rises. When you exhale, notice how the breath drains downwards, away from the upper and the lower part of your lungs, as your belly sinks.

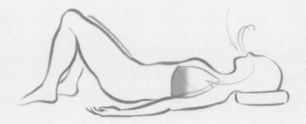

5. On your next inhalation, **breathe only 50 per cent into the lower part of your lungs and pause.** Feel how you are half-full and half-empty

6. Now, inhale the other 50 per cent into the upper part of your lungs. **Pause and feel how full you are.**

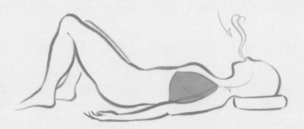

7. **Slowly and gently breathe out through your nose**, releasing the breath completely. Be aware of the emptiness at the end of your out breath. Steps 5–7 count as one complete round. Repeat another 2–4 rounds and then relax your breathing back to its natural flow.

8. On your next exhalation, breathe out just 50 per cent from your upper lungs, **feeling how you are half-full and half-empty**.

Pause and then exhale the remaining 50 per cent from your lower lungs until you are completely empty.

PAUSE AND REST BRIEFLY HERE IN THE EMPTINESS

9. Repeat another 2–4 times, and relax, **letting your breathing flow back into its natural pattern**. Notice any shifts or changes in its quality or feel.

'I would love to
live like a river flows,
carried by the surprise
of its own unfolding.'

JOHN O'DONOHUE

BREATHING TO INDUCE SLEEP

Andrew Weil, a doctor based in Arizona, pioneered this technique. Inspired by yoga's timeless pranayama practices, it has become well known for soothing the nervous system and inducing sleep within minutes. Make sure you are tucked up in bed as you'll be dozing off before you know it.

1. Lying on your back, **rest the tip of your tongue on the roof of your mouth**, on the ridge just behind your upper teeth.

2. Exhale completely and **let your body relax** and sink into the bed.

3. Slowly inhale through your nose for 4 counts and then hold the breath for 7 counts.

NOTE
Slowly build to holding the breath for 7 counts. Holding the breath is not advised for anyone with the conditions listed in our precautions and contraindications section on page 141.

4. On a count of 8, **softly whoosh the breath out** through your mouth, resting your tongue on the floor of your mouth.

5. Continue like this **until sleep prevails.**

'One conscious
breath
– in and out –
is a meditation.'

ECKHART TOLLE

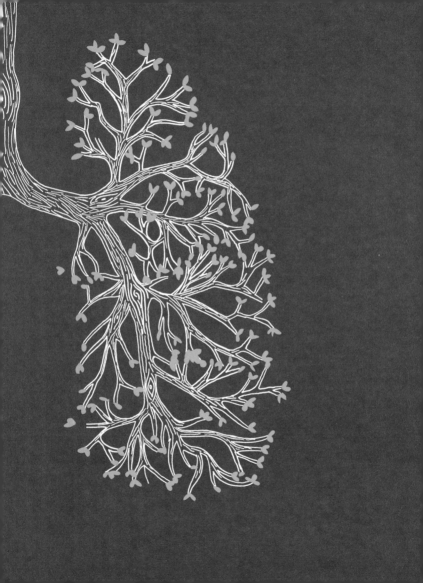

traditional yoga breathing practices

Yoga breathing practices are referred to as 'pranayama', which translates as 'extension of life energy'. The practice of pranayama expands and opens the breath flow throughout the whole body and mind to create clarity, balance and vitality. These are great morning practices and are a wonderful way to super charge your day.

AWAKEN AND ENERGISE (PRANA MUDRA)

This is a simple but powerful practice that connects us to the earth, enabling us to feel its energy (prana) and vitality moving up through our bodies and out again.

1. Sit comfortably on a chair or cushion placed on the ground, in an easy and upright position, as described on page 36. **Anchor through your pelvis and let your crown softly rise.** Rest your hands in your lap, one palm lying on top of the other. Relax and soften your facial muscles and let your eyes close.

2. Become aware of your breath and **let the light of your awareness shine into your breathing.**

IN TURN, SENSE THE **LIGHT** OF YOUR BREATH SHINE INTO YOUR BODY

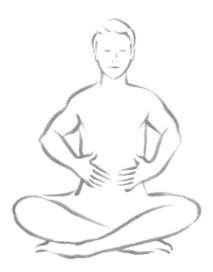

3. On your next inhalation, raise your hands in front of your navel with the fingertips almost touching, **feeling the energy (prana) rising through your body**, as you float your hands up in front of your face.

4. When the in breath is naturally complete, **pause and move your hands apart, opening them up and out in a large V shape**. Let your chest and face softly lift towards the sky.

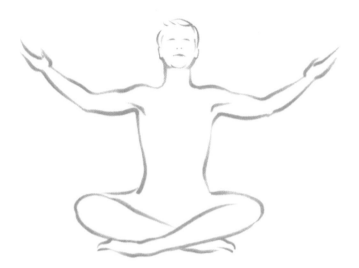

5. Feel your body full of energy (prana) and light **as you breathe in the whole sky**.

6. As you slowly exhale, let go of the sky and bring your breath and arms back down to earth, resting your hands back in your lap. **Pause for a moment to feel the depth of your exhalation** and support of the floor beneath you.

7. This is one complete round. Repeat 5–10 times, then sit quietly for a few moments, **feeling the energy and life flowing within you**.

'Remember, when life's path is steep to keep your mind even.'

HORACE

INNER CLEANSING BREATH (NADI SHODHANA)

This is a traditional yogic breathing practice (pranayama), which helps purify the inner energy channels (nadis) of the body. This aids the flow of energy (prana) through our whole being. It balances the two hemispheres of the brain and is the prefect preparation for meditation.

1. Sit comfortably on a chair or cushion, as described in page 36. **Feel the open length of your spine.**

2. Become aware of your breath and let it settle into a slow and steady rhythm, **inhaling and exhaling fully with each breath.**

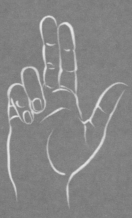

3. **Raise your right hand and bring it into Nose Tip Gesture (Nasagra Mudra)**, placing your index and middle fingers at the space between your eyebrows, your thumb on your right nostril, your ring finger on your left nostril with your little finger softly curled next to your ring finger.

4. Throughout this practice keep your fingers in contact with your nose and **increase and decrease the pressure to modulate the flow of air** in and out of your nostrils.

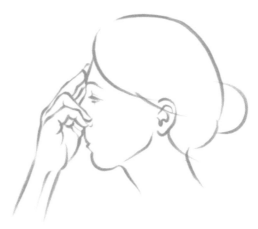

5. **On your next exhalation, relax and release the breath completely.** Then slowly and fully inhale through both nostrils.

6. **Pause as you use your right thumb to close your right nostril.** Slowly, to the count of 5, exhale completely through your left nostril.

7. Once your exhalation is complete, keep the right nostril closed and slowly, to the count of 5, **inhale fully through your left nostril**.

8. **Pause and gently pinch your nose** to close both nostrils.

9. Now release your right thumb slightly to exhale slowly to the count of 5 through your right nostril. **Then inhale fully through your right nostril.**

10. **Pause and gently pinch your nose** to seal both nostrils.

11. This is one complete round. Repeat (from step 6), **alternating the nostrils** for another 4–9 rounds.

12. To finish, calmly rest your hands on your knees and **enjoy a few steady breaths.**

FEELING THE FLOW OF LIFE WITHIN YOU

VICTORIOUS BREATH FOR FOCUS (UJJAYI PRANAYAMA)

This is a traditional yogic technique with a multitude of benefits. The soft, oceanic sound created enables us to hear the flow of our breath, helping to harness and focus the mind. It also generates internal heat that detoxifies the bodily organs and allows muscles and joints to open more efficiently and safely. Perhaps the most noted benefit is that it intensifies the flow of energy throughout the whole body. There are many ways and approaches to this practice: this is just one. Be mindful to keep your face relaxed and the sound of your breath sweet, soft and mellow. No Darth Vader here, please!

1. **Stand tall with ease**, as described on page 39. With your feet hip-width apart, your legs and feet parallel, and the toes pointing forwards, spread your weight evenly across your feet and let the soles open into the ground.

2. **Lengthen along your spine,** allowing your crown to rise and your tail bone to release down. Relax your arms by your sides and soften your shoulders away from your ears.

3. Relax and soften your facial muscles, **let your eyes close and settle here**, becoming aware of your breath.

4. As you inhale through your nose, feel the natural flow of your breath, rising through you as you **breathe in** and washing back down as you **breathe out**.

FEEL ITS FLUID RHYTHM AND ENERGY MOVING
THROUGH YOUR WHOLE BODY

5. **Open your eyes and bring your hands up** approximately 20 cms in front of you, palms facing towards you, elbows bent and soft. Imagine your hands are a mirror.

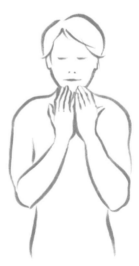

6. Open your mouth slightly, then slowly and fully exhale through your mouth **making a smooth haaaaa sound**, as if you are fogging up a mirror. Let the breath out completely.

7. Inhale through your mouth **creating a soft ahhhhhh sound**, as if defogging the mirror.

8. **Let each breath be full, deep and steady** in both sound and feel.

9. Continue breathing in this way, and **as you inhale, gently sway your weight forwards**, towards your toes, opening your arms up and out to the sides, like wings unfolding.

10. As you exhale, rock your weight back to your heels and **return your hands in front of your mouth to fog the mirror**. If you are seated, you can lean forwards as you inhale and draw back to centre as you exhale.

11. **Feel your chest and heart lifting and opening** with each inhalation, and the belly softly pouring in and up on each exhalation.

NOTE Do not practice this if you have high-blood pressure or any heart conditions

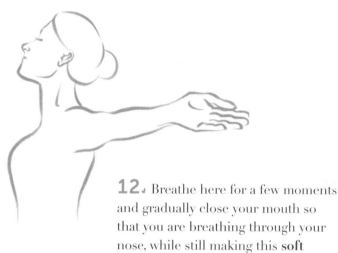

12. Breathe here for a few moments and gradually close your mouth so that you are breathing through your nose, while still making this **soft oceanic** ahhhhhh **sound on the in breath, and** haaaaa **sound on the out breath**.

13. Let the motion of your arms and sway of your body lessen and **slowly diminish so that you are breathing in stillness** with your arms relaxed by your sides.

LISTEN TO THE OCEANIC SOUND OF YOUR BREATH, WASHING THROUGH YOUR BODY

14. Remain here for a few more moments, **enjoying the calm and flow of energy** through your body which *ujjayi* promotes.

' See a world in a
grain of sand
and heaven in a
wild flower,
hold infinity in the
palm of your hand
and eternity in
an hour. '

WILLIAM BLAKE

BELLOWS BREATH AND GLOWING SKULL (BHASTRIKA AND KAPALABHATI)

Both these practices will stoke your inner fire and help to invigorate the abdominal organs, aid digestion and tone the core muscles. *Bhastrika* is a gentler form of *Kapalabhati*, and therefore a good preliminary practice. The practice of *Kapalabhati* improves oxygen circulation through your whole body, particularly to the brain.

BELLOWS BREATH (BHASTRIKA)

1. Come to sit comfortably on a chair or cushion placed on the ground, in an easy and upright position, as described on page 36. **Feel the foundation of your pelvis rooting down.** Softly lengthen through your spine and ease your shoulders down to let your chest open.

2. Place your hands one in front of the other and **turn your palms inwards** to make gentle contact with the lower belly.

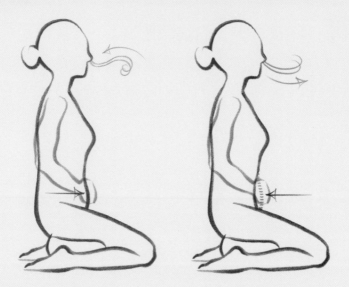

3. Relax and **soften your facial muscles** and let your eyes close.

4. **Enjoy a few steady, deep breaths** and then exhale completely.

5. **Inhale deeply and vigorously**, letting your belly bellow out into your hands.

6. **Exhale with equal strength** and draw your back, in and up, away from your hands.

7. Continue this for another 9 times, **maintaining a steady, even rhythm** with equal inhalations and exhalations. These 10 breaths make one round of *Bhastrika*.

8. Practise another 2–4 rounds and sit quietly, **allowing your breath to return to its natural flow**.

NOTE
When children are taught this practice, it is often called 'stream-train breathing' due to the sound that is made.

GLOWING SKULL (KAPALABHATI)

1. Begin in a comfortable, seated position, as described in *Bhastrika*. **Feel your pelvis rooting into the earth and your spine lengthening up to the sky.** Allow your body to soften and release tension.

2. **Place your palms to rest gently against your lower belly**, with your thumbs level with your navel.

3. **Relax your facial muscles** and let your eyes close.

4. Enjoy a few steady, **deep breaths**.

5. On your next exhalation, **powerfully draw your abdomen in and up, away from your hands**, to expel the breath swiftly.

6. Now release your belly so **the inhalation can pour in without effort**, allowing your belly to make contact with your hands again.

7. Continue this for another 9 times. These **10 breaths make up one round** of *Kapalabhati*.

8. Practice 3–5 rounds, **taking a couple of easy and natural breaths** between each round.

9. To round off the practice, sit quietly with your eyes closed, **allowing your breath to return to its natural flow**, bringing your awareness to your eyebrow centre and feeling an open calmness enveloping your whole body and mind.

NOTE
Bhastrika and *Kapalabhati* should not be practised if pregnant, during menstruation, if you have a hernia, high-blood pressure, lung disease, a gastric ulcer, diarrhoea or if you experience dizziness or anxiety.

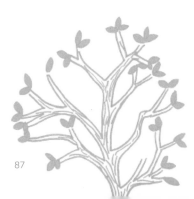

HUMMING BEE
(BHRAMARI PRANAYAMA)

This calming practice helps to soothe and quieten the mind, relax the nervous system, alleviate mental anxiety, tension and anger. The soft vibration created in the throat is considered to be beneficial to singers and public speakers as it lulls the vocal chords and sweetens the voice.

1. **Sit comfortably** on a chair or cushion placed on the ground.

2. Sit in an easy and upright position. **Anchor through your pelvis and softly lengthen your spine**, gently lowering your chin a little.

3. Rest your hands in your lap, **relax and soften your facial muscles and let your eyes close.**

4. Bring your lips together with your teeth slightly parted and your jaw muscles soft. **Settle here and breathe fully and with ease.**

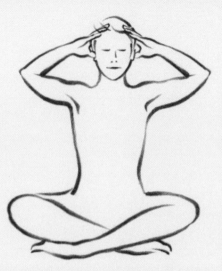

5. **Bring your hands up to your ears** and use your thumbs gently to press the flaps shut while your other fingers rest on top of your head.

6. Keeping your eyes closed, **become aware of the space between the eyebrows,** sometimes referred to as the 'third eye' or 'centre of intuition'.

7. Now **inhale fully** through your nose.

8. Exhale slowly with your mouth closed and **create a soft, smooth, rounded and steady humming sound** that continues to the very end of the out breath. Listen to the sound, feeling the gentle resonation at the front of your skull as the humming flows out. As the hum vibrates through your skull, send the energy down along your spine and let the sound vibrations gently resonate through your whole body.

9. This is one complete round. Repeat 4–7 times. To close the practice, **sit quietly after absorbing the vibrations**.

NOTE
Do not practise this if you are suffering from an ear infection and only do this sitting upright.

' Nature
does not
hurry,

yet everything is
accomplished. '

LAO TZU

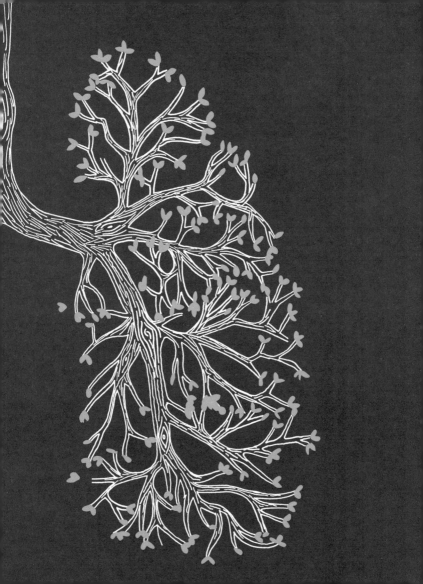

breath-awareness + meditation practices

Breath awareness meditation is not about emptying the mind and thinking of nothing. Instead it gives us time and space to observe our thought patterns as they arise and gain insights to the underlying nature of them and of who we are. Through these practices of breath awareness meditation, we learn to acknowledge our busy mind, thoughts and concerns and to befriend them so that any inner conflict can be calmed and healed.

NATURAL BREATH-
AWARENESS MEDITATION

Breath awareness is at the heart of meditation. It is a way to settle and balance the mind and become present in the moment. Build this practice slowly, starting with just 3 minutes, gradually increasing the duration over time. Some days will feel easier than others, but keep with it and you will reap the benefits for life. Once you have settled into a comfortable sitting position as described on page 36, follow these next four steps to navigate your way to mindful breath-awareness meditation.

1. Soften your eyes and let them close. **Gently bring your mind home to the awareness of your breath**. Without trying to change or shift it, listen to its natural flow and rhythm. Sit here quietly, giving the breath and mind, space and time to settle.

2. In this space, **begin to notice your thoughts as they rise**, calmly watching them without pushing them away, engaging or getting caught up in the drama of them. Simply observe them.

3. Now soften your thinking mind and loosen your grasp on the thoughts, **letting your mind open like a clenched hand slowly unfolding** to release its tight grip.

These first 3 steps may need to be repeated a few times before you feel ready to move on to step 4.

4. As you continue to sit with this awareness of mind and breath, allow your mind to unfurl even more, **opening up like a boundless, cloudless sky.** When thoughts, feelings, plans, regrets and worries arise, as they naturally will, keep returning your mind to the breath, feeling, listening and being aware of your breath to lead you back to the sky like the nature of your mind: **infinite and free.**

BE HERE AND **BREATHE**
WITH YOUR TRUE OPEN NATURE

' We too should
make ourselves
empty, that the
great soul of the
universe may
fill us with
its breath. '

LAURENCE BINYON

BALANCING BREATH

In this practice the flow of your breath is consciously guided in all directions to help lung capacity and cultivate a deep sense of equilibrium and calm within.

1. **Lie down on the floor** in a comfortable position, as described on page 34.

2. Take time to settle, **breathe softly and fully**, relaxing into the natural flow of your breath.

3. As you breathe, sense the cool air entering your nostrils. Gently guide the breath equally in through the right and left nostril and evenly back out again. Take 5 more breaths, **being aware of the flow of air through your nose** on the inhalation and exhalation.

4. Now focus on balancing the length of your in and out breaths, **letting them be easy, relaxed and equal**.

5. Next, bring attention to **balancing the strength of the in and out breaths**, so that one is not more dominant than the other. Take a few breaths here, levelling the length and strength of each inhalation and exhalation.

6. Now gently breathe evenly into the bottom and then into the top of your lungs and back out again (from the top and then the bottom of your lungs). Take a few more breaths here, **feeling the depth and height of your lungs**.

7. Bring awareness to the sides of your torso, breathing evenly into the sides of your lungs, the outer sides by your arms and the inner sides by your spine. **Breathe in and out slowly and gently,** feeling the breadth of your lungs.

8. Widen your attention to the front and back of your body and breathe evenly into the front and back of your lungs. Feel the front and back of your ribcage expand and open with each inhalation and release with each exhalation. **Breathe here, feeling the floor beneath you and the space above you**.

9. Finally, **cultivate an even smoothness** at the beginning and ending of each inhalation and each exhalation.

10. Take a few more breaths here, **enjoying the sense of balance and space** in your body, mind and breath.

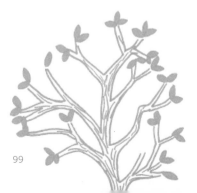

HEART BREATHING

This is a gentle and simple but deeply effective practice that helps to unify breath, heart and mind so that we can operate from a centred place of being. It balances actions from the head and heart.

1. Sit comfortably on a chair or cushion in an easy and upright position. **Feel the stable foundation of your pelvis anchoring down** as you softly lengthen up through your spine. Let your chest open and shoulders relax. Soften your facial muscles and let your eyes close.

2. Place your right hand on your lower belly and feel it gently expanding into your palm as you inhale, and receding as you exhale.

3. Now rest your left hand on your heart. **Feel its beat in your palm** and listen to its rhythm.

4. **Soften your breath and begin to breathe** in time with the beat of your heart. Inhale for 5–6 beats, pause for 1 beat, exhale for 6 beats and pause for 1 beat.

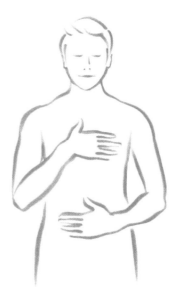

5. Remain here for 5–10 minutes, tuned in to your natural rhythm and **enjoy the synchronicity between your heart and your breath**. Notice your heart's pace on the in breath and on the out breath.

6. When you feel ready, **close the practice by resting both hands over your heart**. Take a few breaths here.

7. Bring your hands together and **rub your palms to generate heat in your hands**. When they feel warm, lightly place your palms over your eyelids.

FEEL THE **WARM** DARKNESS ENVELOPING YOU

With your palms still in the same position, **gradually open your eyes and begin to move your hands away** and down to your lap, as your eyes adjust to the light around you.

' There is one
way of breathing
that is shameful
and constricted.

Then, there's is another
way: a breath of love
that takes you all the
way to infinity. '

RUMI

RECOVERING THE HEART (ANAHATA)

Sometimes we may feel disconnected from our feelings and emotions due to past hurt or traumas. This can cause our hearts to feel tight and closed. This calming practice helps to reopen and heal our hearts so that we can restore to our life a sense of warmth and understanding.

1. Sit comfortably on a chair or cushion placed on the ground and **feel your pelvis rooting to the ground**. Softly lengthen up through your spine and gently ease your shoulders back and down to help open your chest.

2. **Become aware of your breath** and allow it to flow slowly and fully deep into your body, softly expanding and opening as you inhale, and gently releasing and relaxing as you exhale.

3. As your breath becomes steady and easy, direct your awareness to your heart. Have a sense of its shape, weight and feeling. **Breathe into your heart and listen. Breathe out from your heart and soften.** Take a few breaths here.

4. Now, with deepened awareness, send your breath to your heart and let it open and expand as you inhale. **As you exhale allow your heart to soften and yield**, letting the hard edges melt away and any hurt, pain, grudge or resentment to dissolve and release.

5. To enhance this practice, bring your hands into *Hridaya Mudra* (heart gesture) by softly curling your index finger under your thumb, placing the tips of the middle and ring fingers on the tip of your thumb and extending your little finger. This directs the flow of energy from the hands to the heart, **to open, unburden, fortify and strengthen its physical and emotional state.**

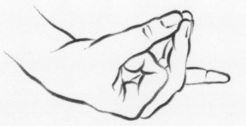

BREATH AWARENESS
TO RELEASE ANXIETY

The following meditation helps to level and calm the breath, soothing the mind and releasing any anxiety and tension in the body.

1. Sit comfortably on a chair or cushion as described on page 36. Sit in an easy and upright position. **Relax, soften your facial muscles and let your eyes close** and settle here.

2. **Become aware of your breath and notice how you are breathing**, without changing anything. Are you breathing through your nose, mouth or both? How does your breath feel? It is short or long? Is it shallow or deep? Take a few breaths and accept the breath for how it is. **LETTING IT BE**

3. On your next exhalation breathe out completely. **Gently, inhale deeply through your nose**, feeling when you are full and then softly exhaling through your mouth, emptying your lungs completely and sighing out.

4. Repeat 2–4 times, **letting your mind and body soften** on each out breath.

5. Now let your breath flow steadily through your nose. **Allow each out breath to come to its natural end**, and then gently open to each in breath.

6. When your attention moves away from your breath and begins to focus on other things, observe that this has happened and **be aware of what you are thinking and feeling**. Simply notice the thoughts and accompanying feelings that arise. Notice the physical changes without altering anything. Can you watch what happens? Can you observe your own thoughts and feelings? Be aware that these thoughts and feelings are a natural response to the situation you find yourself in.

LET YOURSELF SOFTEN AND ACCEPT YOUR FEELINGS WITH EACH **BREATH**

7. Gently bring your attention back to your breath and its flow. **Breathe in and out fully and completely,** letting each breath come to its natural and complete end.

8. **Each time your mind wanders, notice this and witness the thoughts and feelings.** Breathe with them and know that they are not you. Gently bring your awareness back to the natural flow of your breath.

RIDE EACH BREATH, THOUGHT
AND FEELING LIKE A SURFER
RIDES A WAVE, LETTING THEM
RISE AND THEN FALL AWAY

' A thought is harmless
unless we believe it.

It's not our thoughts,
but our attachment
to our thoughts, that
causes suffering. '

BYRON KATIE

WALKING BREATH-AWARENESS MEDITATION

The body loves the natural momentum of walking. It is part of our evolution. This love can easily be tapped into and rediscovered. This is a lovely practice to do barefoot on any surface – grass, sand or wooden floors.

1. **Begin quietly by standing with your attention resting on your breath.** Feel its sensation moving through your body as your feet release into the ground.

2. With ease, start walking, allowing your stride to be natural, following the steps on page 112. **Go slowly without haste, letting your eyeline be level and your focus soft and open.** Sense and absorb everything around you.

3. **As you walk, feel your feet making easy and deep contact with the ground.** Notice how your feet roll from heel to the toe. Be aware of the shift of weight from one foot to the other, the soft swing of your arms, the length at the back of your neck and the flow of your breath.

' As we walk,

imprint our
gratitude and
our love to
the earth. '

THICH NHAT HANH

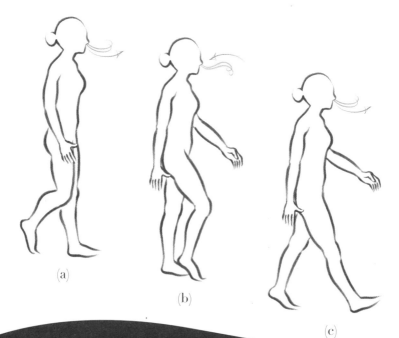

(a)

(b)

(c)

WALKING BREATH

(a) Exhale, planting your **LEFT** foot down (heel first) into the ground, rolling through the foot (ball and toes) as the body's weight moves forwards.

(b) Inhale, floating the **RIGHT** knee forwards, bringing the foot through.

4. Become aware of your whole body as one foot steps in front of the other. **Allow your breathing to fall in rhythm with your steps**, easily and slowly.

5. **Let your mind be aware of each step,** each breath and each moment. Continue in this way for 10–20 minutes.

6. To finish, stand quietly for a few moments, as you did at the start, **enjoying this moment of calm**.

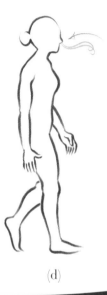

(d)

(c) Exhale, taking another step forwards with your **LEFT** foot, planting the foot down (heel first, then ball and toe) into the ground.

(d) Inhale, floating the **RIGHT** knee forwards.

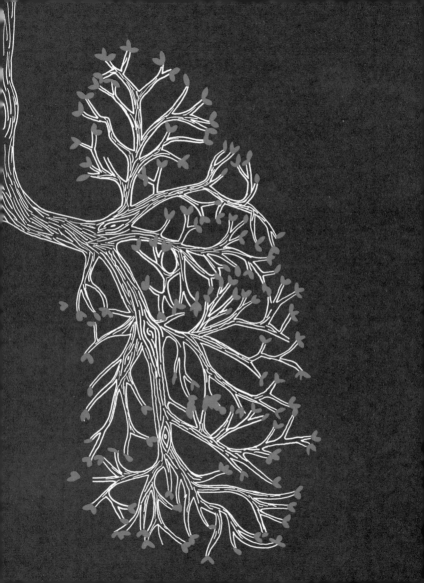

breath-inspired movement practices

The breath is movement and is the link between the body and the mind. The more aware we become of our breath's flow, the more we are able to tap into the breath's energy to carry, support and inspire the body's movement, helping to bring the breathing body and mind together, to move as one in harmony into a flowing movement meditation.

AWAKENING THE SPINE

This practice is traditionally referred to as *Bitilasana* and *Marjariasana*, meaning 'cow' and 'cat' pose. It tones the abdomen, warms up the back muscles and articulates the spine. It also expands and opens the front and back of the lungs, harmonising the flow of breath with the motion of the body.

1. **Begin on all-fours**, placing your hands directly under your shoulders and your knees under your hips, so that your arms and thighs are perpendicular to the floor.

2. **Lengthen your arms, and softly spread your palms down into the floor**, with your fingers fanning apart and the index fingers pointing forwards.

3. **Curl your toes**, yielding them to the floor.

4. Bring awareness to your back and lengthen your spine from crown to tail bone, **creating a coffee-table shape with your back**.

5. Exhale and **let the breath flow out**.

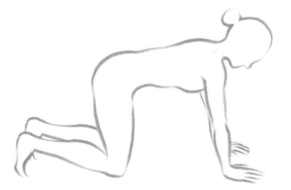

6. On your next inhalation, gently extend your crown forwards, as you lift your face and open the heart. At the same time, extend your tail bone backwards and up, tilting your pelvis, **creating a soft curve or smile through the length of your spine**.

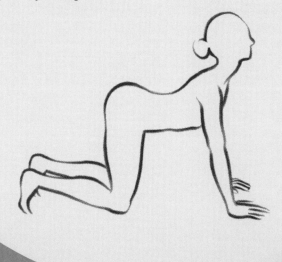

NOTE
If you are pregnant, avoid scooping in your belly. Keep the abdomen loose. For those people with any disc displacement or Diastrasis Recti, avoid curling or arching your back, maintaining a flat back instead while drawing in the abdomen inwards and upwards.

7. On your next exhalation, round your spine and scoop in your belly to expand and **mushroom your back upwards in the opposite direction.** Release your head and hips downwards.

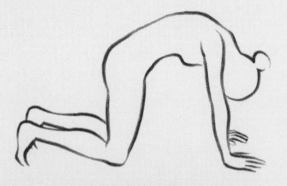

8. This is one complete round. **Continue in this way, moving your spine up and down to the flow of your breath** for another 6–9 times.

9. To finish, gently draw your hips back onto your heels and rest your forehead on the ground, **relaxing your body and listening to your breath.**

STREAMLINE FLOOR FLOW

This is fluid exercise will cultivates grace and ease of movement, and develops length and extension throughout the body while having the support of the ground.

1. Lie down on the floor in a comfortable position, as described on page 34. **Release and enjoy the support of the ground beneath you**. Settle here letting your breath flow softly, deeply and naturally.

2. When you feel ready, inhale and stretch long, reaching your arms out by the sides of your head and your legs, away from your fingertips. **Streamline and breathe through your whole body**.

RELISH THE FEELING OF...

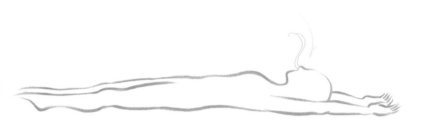

3. On your next exhalation bend your right leg, taking your hands to your right knee. Softly hug and ease the right knee down towards your body. **Let the breath empty completely from your lungs.**

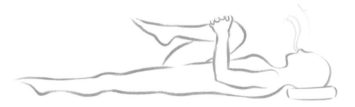

...OPENNESS AND LENGTH

4. On your next inhalation, lower your right leg and stretch it long into the floor. **Streamline your body as the breath flows into all your limbs,** fingers and toes, reaching away. As your inhalation completes, fill your body with energy.

5. **On your next exhalation,** bend and hug your left leg.

6. Continue to move with your breath in this way a few more times. Let it be a fluid experience, opening and **lengthening as you breathe in, then softening and hugging one leg as you breathe out**.

7. After 10–20 times, rest your body, releasing into the floor **like a relaxed, happy starfish basking in the sun.**

'Movement is the
song of the body.'

VANDA SCARAVELLI

CLEARING INNER SPACE

This is a Qigong practice that I learned from my good colleague Mimi Kuo Deemer. It is a gentle but powerful clearing technique that combines simple movement with breath and mindful intention to release negativity and welcome positivity.

1. **Stand and plant your feet into the ground** a little wider than hip-width apart, with your legs and feet parallel and your toes pointing forwards. Soften your knees, relax your belly and bring your pelvis in line with your feet. Place your arms by your sides.

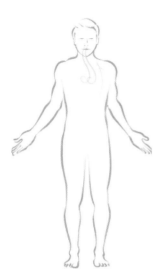

2. On your next inhalation, **breathe length into your spine** and release your arms and shoulders down, with your palms turned up as if allowing a butterfly to rest on each one. Take a few steady and full breaths here.

3. On your next inhalation, slowly raise your arms up and out, **gathering the feelings, qualities, emotions, belief systems and patterns** that no longer serve you but hold you back or make you doubt yourself. Recognise what they are and draw them up to the sky.

4. On your next exhalation, turn your palms down, lowering your arms in front of you, and softly bend your knees. **Consciously release these gathered feelings down and out into the earth.** Let them flow through and out of you on your out breath.

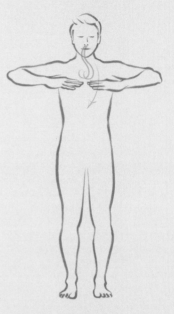

5. Repeat this 2 more times, **mindfully gathering and clearing**.

6. On your next inhalation, while raising your arms, **gather positive qualities, feelings, emotions and thought patterns**. Acknowledge and feel what they are as you gather them.

7. On your next exhalation, as you lower your arms, let those qualities flow into you and fill the inner space. **Feel the sensation of these qualities deep in your core.**

8. Repeat this 2 more times, **mindfully gathering and filling**.

9. On your next inhalation, gather these positive feelings and emotions once again, as you **raise your arms to the sky**.

10. Lower your arms with a slow, steady exhalation and seal these qualities deep within the inner space of your being. **Feel the existence of them in your core.**

11. Repeat this 2 more times, breathing with **clear, conscious intention**.

12. To close this practice, **breathe and stand quietly for a few moments**, absorbing the benefits of this exercise and nurturing the positive qualities within you.

ELEMENTAL BREATHING:
PART 1

In our bodies we replicate the most fundamental elements of this planet – earth, fire, water, air and ether. At different times any of the elements may dominate and affect our energetic, mental and emotional states. The following two practices are designed to restore balance to these inner elements.

1. Begin standing tall with your feet hip-width apart as described on page 39. **Let the soles of your feet open into the ground and spread your weight evenly.** Softly lengthen up through your spine and feel your crown floating upwards to create a sense of openness and space in your body. Rest your arms down by your sides, with your shoulders relaxing back and down.

2. Relax and soften your facial muscles, let your eyes close and become aware of your breath. Listen to its natural flow and rhythm. **Feel the energy rising through your body as you inhale** and descending as you exhale. Settle and fully immerse your awareness in your breath.

3. Exhale completely, and on your next inhalation, open your eyes and arms out to the side, palms facing up. **Continue raising your arms as the breath rises and fills.** When the inhalation is complete, bring your hands together over your head, palm to palm.

4. **Exhale slowly, softly bending your knees.** Keeping your fingertips in contact, part your palms, bringing them down in front of your face. Lower your hands back down by your sides.

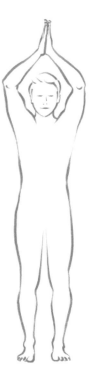

5. This is one complete round. **Repeat, seeing the breath as warm light as you inhale, rising through your body as you inhale**, like sunlight filling a room. When you exhale, feel the breath as warm water or monsoon rain gently washing down through your body. Repeat 6 times.

6. Close this practice by standing and **breathing for a few moments** with your eyes closed.

FEEL YOUR WHOLE BODY
BEING DRENCHED IN THE
FLOW OF YOUR BREATH

'Who looks
outside
dreams,

who looks
inside
awakens'

CARL JUNG

' Walk tall as the trees,
live strong as the mountains
Be gentle as the spring winds,

Keep the warmth of the
summer sun in your heart
and the great spirit
will always be with you. '

NATIVE AMERICAN PROVERB

ELEMENTAL BREATHING: PART 2

1. Follow steps 1 and 2 of the previous practice.

2. As you inhale, **raise the right arm only**.

3. On your next exhalation, gently reach the right hand overhead to the left side of your body, **the body leaning over like a tree yielding to the wind**, but remaining rooted.

4. Inhale and feel the right side of your body **lengthening and opening**.

5. On your next exhalation, bend your knees and gently roll your torso around and down over your legs, folding at the hips. Fully inhale and exhale here with your arms, shoulders, neck and **head hanging down like a rag doll**. Allow your knees to soften.

6. On your next inhalation, bend your knees and **slowly roll up through your spine** to a standing position.

EXHALE FULLY

7. Repeat steps 3–6 but **raise your left arm as you inhale**.

8. Take a few breaths, feeling centred as you stand. **Sense the earth beneath you offering support** as the breath flows through you.

9. Now try 3 complete rounds of part 1 followed by part 2 on both sides of your body. At the end, take 5 slow breaths, **enjoying the feeling of fluidity and the sense of earth beneath your feet**, space above your crown and air around your body.

HALF SUN SALUTATIONS

Sun Salutations are a traditional yoga practice. They are a wonderful way to start the day, waking up the body and mind and greeting new energy. However, they can be practised any time to rejuvenate your whole being.

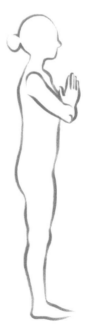

1. Stand with your feet together or apart. Choose what makes you feel most grounded and centred. **Let the soles of your feet breathe into the ground** and gently lengthen your spine. Be spacious and easy. Rest your hands, palm to palm, in front of your chest.

2. Let your eyes close and become aware of your breath. Feel its natural energy, opening and expanding within you when you inhale, **releasing tiredness and tension as you exhale.**

TAKE A FEW BREATHS

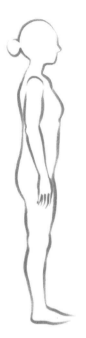

3. On your next exhalation, **release your arms down by your sides** and open your eyes.

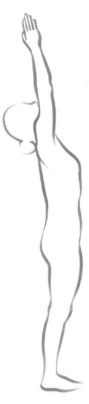

4. Breathe in and float your **arms out to the sides** and up over your head, bringing your hands together, palm to palm.

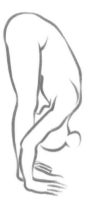

5. Exhale fully, bending your knees and folding forwards from your hips. If it feels comfortable, straighten your legs, otherwise keep them bent. **At the same time, sweep your arms out to your sides, like wings soaring open as you bow low to the earth.** Place your hands on the floor and rest your front ribs on your thighs.

6. **Inhale along the length of your spine**, lift your heart and extend your back so it is parallel to the ground. Keep your knees bent.

7. Exhale fully, **releasing your body down and over your legs again**. Relax your arms, shoulders and neck muscles so that your head drops down. If it feels comfortable, straighten your legs.

8. On your next inhalation, **slowly uncurl back to standing**, feeling your feet rooting down as your arms open up above, returning the palms together, saluting the sky.

9. Breathe out and softly swim your arms back down to your sides, standing tall and easy. This is one complete Sun Salutation.

10. Repeat another 5 times, **letting the breath lead your body** to create fluidity of movement.

11. To finish, stand quietly. Notice the energy (prana) flowing through your body with each breath. **Sense the ground beneath and the sky above.** Allow yourself to balance between these two great elements. Feel how these two natural forces meet and flow within you.

'Take my hand.
We will walk.
We will only walk.
We will enjoy
our walk
without
thinking of
arriving
anyway. '

THICH NHAT HANH

SAFETY NOTES

Although breathing is completely safe (if not essential!)
there are important points to observe that help enhance
the breath and safeguard against any medical conditions
being exacerbated by the breathing practices outlined in
this book.

To reap the benefits from the practices, please read
through this list before embarking on any of them.

- Never strain or force your breath.
- Listen to your breathing.
- Do not rush.
- Take time to connect to your breath, feeling the sensation
  of your breath flowing through your body.
- Relax and close your eyes through the practices to help
  deepen your awareness of your breath.
- If possible, always breathe through your nose on the in and
  out breaths unless otherwise instructed.
- At the end of each practice take your time to rest and
  absorb the benefits, then consciously note you have
  completed the practice before moving slowly and gently
  into your daily activities.
- If you experience discomfort or unease in any of the
  practices, take a few moments to open your eyes and sit
  quietly before re-entering the practice or finishing it.

Do not hold or retain the breath if you have been diagnosed with any of the conditions listed below.

- Coronary disease
- Hypertension
- Aneurysm
- Hernia
- Gastric ulcer
- Recent abdominal or thoracic surgery
- Abdominal, pelvic, retinal, pulmonary disease
- Bipolar disorder
- Schizophrenia
- Dissociative disorder
- Anxiety
- Epilepsy
- Stroke
- Pregnancy
- Lung cancer
- Lung disease
- Asthma
- Chronic bronchitis

If you have any of the above, are recovering from any type of surgery or have any medical condition/s or concerns, it is essential that you check with your doctor before practising any of the exercises contained within this book.

The author has made every effort to ensure all the instructions in this book are safe and accurate. However, it is necessary to always seek medical advice if you have any concerns about your suitability for any of the breathing practices in this book, as the author and publishers can not accept liability for any resulting injury, or damage to persons or property, however it may arise. This book does not replace medical consultation and should be used in conjunction with professional advice.

QUOTES WERE TAKEN FROM:

Byron Katie is an American speaker and author.

Carl Jung was a Swiss psychiatrist and psychotherapist.

Clarissa Pinkola Estes is an American Jungian analyst and author.

Erkhart Tolle is a German-born public speaker and spiritual teacher, best known for his bestseller *The Power of Now*.

John O'Donohue was an poet, priest and Hegelian philosopher

Horace was the leading Roman lyric writer.

Lao Tzu was a philosopher and author of *Tao Te Ching*.

Laurence Binyon was an English poet, dramatist and art scholar.

Rumi was Persian poet and Sufi master born in 1207.

Thich Nhat Hanh is a Vietnamese Zen Buddist monk, author and peace activist.

Vanda Scaravelli made a profound impact on hatha yoga. Her book, *Awakening the Spine* has become a classic.

William Blake was a 19th Century writer and artist. He is regarded as a seminal figure of the Romantic Age.

With thanks to Felix, for being my eternal inspiration, and to John and Val for their ceaseless support.

Publishing Director Sarah Lavelle
Creative Director Helen Lewis
Editor Harriet Butt
Copy Editor Victoria Marshallsay
Designer Nicola Ellis
Cover Design and Illustration Emily Lapworth
Illustrator Juliet Percival
Production Emily Noto, Vincent Smith

First published in 2016 by
Quadrille Publishing
Pentagon House
52–54 Southwark Street
London SE1 1UN
www.quadrille.co.uk
www.quadrille.com

Quadrille is an imprint of
Hardie Grant
www.hardiegrant.com.au

Text © 2016 Jean Hall
All instructional illustrations
© 2016 Juliet Purcival
Artwork, design and layout
© 2016 Quadrille Publishing Ltd

Cataloguing in Publication Data: a catalogue record for this book is available from the British Library.

ISBN: 978 184949 774 9

Printed in China

Citation for the quote used on page 14: Estés, Ph.D., Clarissa Pinkola, Women Who Run with the Wolves: Contacting the Power of the Wild Woman. (Rider, 2008), p. 160, with kind permission of author and publisher.